THE SOLUTION FOR BLOOD SUGAR

The Blueprint for Balancing Blood Sugar and Transforming Your Health

Timothy Deberry

Disclaimer

The contents of this book are intended for informational and entertainment purposes only. While every effort has been made to ensure the accuracy and completeness of the information provided, the author and publisher make no representations or warranties, express or implied, about the completeness, accuracy, reliability, suitability, or availability with respect to the content contained within these pages.

The information contained in this book is not intended to serve as professional advice or guidance. Readers are encouraged to consult with appropriate professionals or experts in their respective fields for specific advice tailored to their individual circumstances.

The author and publisher shall not be liable for any loss, damage, or injury arising from the use or reliance on the information contained in this book. Any reliance you place on such information is strictly at your own risk.

All opinions expressed in this book are those of the author and do not necessarily reflect the views of the publisher. Reference to specific products, services, companies, or individuals does not imply endorsement or recommendation by the author or publisher, unless explicitly stated.

The inclusion of any links or references to external websites does not imply endorsement or approval of the content, products, services, or opinions offered by those websites.

Readers are advised to use their discretion and judgment when implementing any suggestions or recommendations provided in this book. Ultimately, the responsibility for any actions taken based on the information in this book lies solely with the reader.

Copyright © 2024. All rights reserved.

Table of Contents

DISCLAIMER.. 2

INTRODUCTION.. 8

UNVEILING THE BLOOD SUGAR SOLUTION 8

THE SIGNIFICANCE OF BLOOD SUGAR................................ 8
OVERVIEW OF THE BLOOD SUGAR SOLUTION 8

CHAPTER 1 11

UNDERSTANDING BLOOD SUGAR 11

BASICS OF BLOOD SUGAR (GLUCOSE) 11
THE IMPACT OF IMBALANCED BLOOD SUGAR 12

CHAPTER 2 14

FACTORS AFFECTING BLOOD SUGAR LEVELS 14

DIET AND NUTRITION.. 14
PHYSICAL ACTIVITY 15
STRESS AND ITS INFLUENCE ON BLOOD SUGAR 15

CHAPTER 3 17

THE BLOOD SUGAR SOLUTION LIFESTYLE 17

DIETARY GUIDELINES 17

EXERCISE AND PHYSICAL ACTIVITY 18
STRESS REDUCTION TECHNIQUES 18

CHAPTER 4 .... **20**

**MONITORING AND MANAGING BLOOD SUGAR
LEVELS** **20**

BLOOD GLUCOSE MONITORING **20**
MEDICATIONS AND SUPPLEMENTS 21
LIFESTYLE STRATEGIES FOR EFFECTIVE MANAGEMENT 21

CHAPTER 5 .... **23**

MEAL PLANNING AND RECIPES **23**

MEAL PLANS FOR BLOOD SUGAR CONTROL 23
14-DAY MEAL PLAN FOR BLOOD SUGAR CONTROL 24
HEALTHY RECIPES TAILORED FOR BLOOD SUGAR BALANCE
.... 36
RECIPES **37**

CHAPTER 6 .... **51**

OVERCOMING CHALLENGES **51**

DEALING WITH SUGAR CRAVINGS 51
DINING OUT STRATEGIES 52
NAVIGATING RESTAURANT CHALLENGES: 52
NAVIGATING SOCIAL EVENTS AND HOLIDAYS 52

CHAPTER 7 .... **54**

LONG-TERM HEALTH AND WELLNESS **54**

PREVENTION OF TYPE 2 DIABETES 54
BLOOD SUGAR SOLUTION FOR WEIGHT MANAGEMENT 55
IMPACT ON OVERALL HEALTH AND WELL-BEING 55

CHAPTER 8 .... **57**

REAL-LIFE SUCCESS STORIES **57**

PERSONAL JOURNEYS TO BLOOD SUGAR CONTROL 57
LESSONS LEARNED AND INSPIRATIONAL NARRATIVES 58
ENCOURAGEMENT FOR YOUR JOURNEY 58

CHAPTER 9 .... **60**

RESOURCES FOR FURTHER SUPPORT **60**

BOOKS AND READING MATERIALS 60
IN-DEPTH KNOWLEDGE: 60
WORKSHOPS AND SEMINARS 61
ONLINE COMMUNITIES AND FORUMS 62
PROFESSIONAL GUIDANCE 62

CHAPTER 10 .... **64**

EMBRACING A LIFE OF BALANCED BLOOD SUGAR **64**

RECAP OF KEY POINTS 64
ENCOURAGEMENT FOR THE JOURNEY AHEAD 65
WISHING YOU A HAPPY AND FULFILLING FUTURE **66**

CONCLUSION **68**

Introduction
Unveiling The Blood Sugar Solution

Here's to reaching the ideal blood sugar balance and living a happier, healthier life—with "The Blood Sugar Solution". The significant influence that blood sugar levels have on our overall health is sometimes overlooked in our fast-paced, convenience-driven society. Your road map to comprehending, controlling, and becoming an expert at preserving stable blood sugar levels is this book.

The Significance of Blood Sugar

The fundamental component of all of our body's complex systems is glucose. This seemingly uncomplicated molecule is essential to our daily existence since it provides our cells with energy required for our daily survival. But the fine balance of blood sugar is susceptible to disruption, which can result in a host of health challenges which can affect not just our physical health but also our mental health.

Overview of The Blood Sugar Solution

"The Blood Sugar Solution" is not just a book—it's a holistic approach to wellness, a lifestyle shift that empowers you to take control of your health. Whether you're aiming to prevent diabetes, manage your weight, or simply enhance your overall vitality, this guide is tailored to provide you with the knowledge, tools, and practical strategies needed to achieve and maintain balanced blood sugar levels.

In the chapters that follow, we will delve into the intricacies of blood sugar regulation, explore the factors influencing its balance, and uncover a comprehensive solution that encompasses nutrition, physical activity, stress management, and more. This is not a one-size-fits-all approach; instead, it is a personalized journey that recognizes the uniqueness of each individual's body and lifestyle.

Through real-life success stories, practical meal plans, and actionable tips, "The Blood Sugar Solution" will equip you with the tools to make informed choices about your health. Whether you're at the beginning of your wellness journey or seeking to enhance your current lifestyle, this guide is designed to meet you where you are and guide you toward a future of sustained well-being.

As we embark on this journey together, remember that small, consistent changes can lead to remarkable transformations. Your commitment to understanding and managing your blood sugar is an investment in your present and future health, and this guide is here to support you every step of the way.

Get ready to unravel the mysteries of blood sugar, embrace a lifestyle that fosters balance, and witness the positive impact it can have on your overall health and vitality. Let "The Blood Sugar Solution" be your companion on the path to a healthier, happier, and more energized you. Here's to your journey to optimal blood sugar and a life of well-being!

Chapter 1
Understanding Blood Sugar

Welcome to the foundational chapter of "The Blood Sugar Solution." In this segment, we'll embark on a journey to unravel the intricacies of blood sugar—what it is, why it matters, and how it influences our daily lives. By gaining a deeper understanding of this vital aspect of our physiology, you'll be better equipped to navigate the path towards balanced blood sugar and enhanced well-being.

Basics of Blood Sugar (Glucose)

Role in the Body:

At its core, blood sugar, or glucose, serves as the primary fuel for our body's cells. Imagine it as the energy currency that powers our daily activities, from the most basic cellular functions to the vigorous demands of physical exercise. Understanding its central role in our body's energy production is crucial to appreciating the significance of maintaining an optimal balance.

Regulation Mechanisms:

The body operates with precision, continuously regulating blood sugar levels to ensure they stay within a narrow range. Organs such as the pancreas and the liver play pivotal roles in this intricate dance. Insulin, a hormone produced by the pancreas, facilitates the absorption of glucose into cells, while the liver stores and releases glucose as needed. This delicate interplay maintains stability, but disruptions can lead to both short-term and long-term health consequences.

The Impact of Imbalanced Blood Sugar

Short-Term Effects:

When blood sugar levels swing too high or too low, the body responds with noticeable signals. Symptoms of high blood sugar may include increased thirst, frequent urination, and fatigue. On the flip side, low blood sugar can manifest as irritability, dizziness, and confusion. Recognizing these signs is crucial for proactive management.

Long-Term Health Consequences:

Prolonged imbalances in blood sugar levels can give rise to serious health issues. The risk of developing conditions such as Type 2 diabetes, cardiovascular disease, and other metabolic disorders increases when blood sugar is consistently elevated. This chapter will shed light on the importance of preventing and managing these long-term consequences through informed lifestyle choices.

As we delve into the intricacies of blood sugar, consider this chapter as the cornerstone of your journey toward optimal health. Armed with the knowledge of its fundamental role and the impact of imbalances, you are now better prepared to explore the factors influencing blood sugar levels and the actionable steps to achieve balance in the chapters that follow.

Chapter 2
Factors Affecting Blood Sugar Levels

Now that we've laid the groundwork for understanding blood sugar, it's time to explore the dynamic interplay of factors that influence its delicate balance. In this chapter, we'll delve into the multifaceted aspects of our daily lives that impact blood sugar levels, empowering you with insights to make informed choices and cultivate a lifestyle that fosters stability.

Diet and Nutrition

Impact of Carbohydrates:

Carbohydrates play a pivotal role in blood sugar regulation. Different types of carbohydrates affect blood sugar levels differently. Simple carbohydrates, found in sugary foods, can cause rapid spikes, while complex carbohydrates, found in whole grains and vegetables, release glucose more gradually. Understanding these distinctions allows you to make mindful choices that promote sustained energy and stable blood sugar levels.

Role of Proteins and Fats:

Proteins and fats also influence blood sugar regulation. Combining carbohydrates with protein and healthy fats can slow down the absorption of glucose, mitigating spikes. This chapter will provide insights into crafting balanced meals that promote optimal blood sugar control.

Physical Activity

Exercise and Blood Sugar Regulation:

Physical activity is a powerful tool for managing blood sugar levels. Regular exercise enhances insulin sensitivity, allowing cells to more effectively absorb glucose. We'll explore the types and intensity of exercises that can positively impact blood sugar, as well as strategies to incorporate movement into your daily routine.

Sedentary Lifestyle's Effect on Blood Sugar:

Conversely, a sedentary lifestyle can contribute to imbalances in blood sugar. Prolonged periods of inactivity may lead to insulin resistance, hindering the body's ability to regulate glucose effectively. Discover how even small increments of movement can make a significant difference in maintaining blood sugar stability.

Stress and Its Influence on Blood Sugar

Cortisol and Blood Sugar Levels:

The stress hormone cortisol can have a profound impact on blood sugar levels. During stressful situations, the body releases glucose to provide immediate energy for the "fight or flight" response. Chronic stress, however, can lead to sustained elevated blood sugar. Learn effective stress management techniques to mitigate its impact on your blood sugar.

Stress Management Techniques:

Explore mindfulness, meditation, and relaxation exercises as powerful tools to manage stress levels. Integrating these practices into your daily life can contribute not only to emotional well-being but also to balanced blood sugar levels.

As we navigate the factors affecting blood sugar, consider this chapter as a guide to making intentional choices in your diet, physical activity, and stress management. By understanding how these elements influence blood sugar levels, you'll be better equipped to adopt a lifestyle that supports your journey toward optimal health and well-being.

Chapter 3
The Blood Sugar Solution Lifestyle

In this pivotal chapter, we transition from understanding the intricacies of blood sugar to crafting a lifestyle that nurtures its delicate balance. The Blood Sugar Solution Lifestyle is not a temporary fix but a holistic approach designed to become an integral part of your everyday routine. Let's explore the key pillars of this transformative lifestyle that will empower you to take charge of your health and well-being.

Dietary Guidelines

Low Glycemic Foods:

The foundation of The Blood Sugar Solution Lifestyle lies in embracing a diet rich in low-glycemic foods. These foods release glucose gradually, preventing sudden spikes and crashes in blood sugar levels. This chapter will guide you in making informed choices, incorporating whole grains, vegetables, and other low-glycemic options into your meals.

Balanced Meals and Snacks:

The timing and composition of meals play a crucial role in blood sugar regulation. Discover the art of crafting balanced meals and snacks that combine carbohydrates, proteins, and healthy fats to promote sustained energy and stable blood sugar levels throughout the day.

Exercise and Physical Activity

Effective Workout Strategies:

Engaging in regular physical activity is a cornerstone of The Blood Sugar Solution Lifestyle. Learn about effective workout strategies that not only boost your overall well-being but also enhance insulin sensitivity, facilitating better blood sugar control.

Incorporating Movement into Daily Life:

Exercise doesn't have to be confined to the gym. Explore creative ways to incorporate movement into your daily life, whether through walking, cycling, or simple at-home exercises. These small but consistent efforts can make a significant impact on your blood sugar levels.

Stress Reduction Techniques

Mindfulness and Meditation:

The practice of mindfulness and meditation holds profound benefits for both mental well-being and blood sugar control. Discover simple yet powerful techniques that can help you navigate stress and cultivate a sense of calm in your daily life.

Relaxation Exercises:

Incorporate relaxation exercises into your routine to counteract the impact of stress on blood sugar levels. Techniques such as deep breathing and progressive muscle relaxation can become valuable tools in maintaining balance. As you immerse yourself in The Blood Sugar Solution Lifestyle, consider this chapter as a blueprint for sustainable, positive change. By integrating these guidelines into your daily routine, you'll not only support optimal blood sugar levels but also enhance your overall health and vitality. Get ready to embrace a lifestyle that empowers you to thrive, one balanced blood sugar level at a time.

Chapter 4
Monitoring and Managing Blood Sugar Levels

As we journey deeper into "The Blood Sugar Solution," we now turn our attention to the vital aspect of monitoring and managing blood sugar levels. Armed with knowledge and insights, you'll gain the tools to actively participate in your well-being, ensuring that your blood sugar remains in balance. In this chapter, we'll explore the importance of regular monitoring, interpret readings, and delve into various strategies for effective management.

Blood Glucose Monitoring

Importance of Regular Monitoring:

Regular monitoring of blood sugar levels is a cornerstone of proactive health management. Understanding the significance of consistent monitoring empowers you to track trends, identify patterns, and make informed decisions about your lifestyle choices. This chapter will guide you on how and when to monitor your blood sugar effectively.

Interpreting Blood Glucose Readings:

Blood glucose readings are not just numbers—they are valuable insights into your body's response to various factors. Learn to interpret your readings, recognizing patterns of highs and lows, and gaining a deeper understanding of how different aspects of your lifestyle impact blood sugar levels.

Medications and Supplements

Prescription Medications:

For some individuals, medication may be a part of their blood sugar management plan. Explore common prescription medications, their mechanisms, and how they work to maintain blood sugar stability. Always consult with your healthcare provider for personalized guidance.

Herbal and Nutritional Supplements:

Complementary to traditional medications, certain herbal and nutritional supplements may offer additional support in managing blood sugar levels. Discover the potential benefits of supplements and how they can be integrated into a holistic approach to blood sugar control.

Lifestyle Strategies for Effective Management

Dietary Adjustments:

Building on the dietary guidelines discussed in previous chapters, learn how specific dietary adjustments can be tailored to your blood sugar management needs. Explore the impact of portion control, meal timing, and mindful eating practices on maintaining stability.

Exercise as a Management Tool:

Physical activity is not only a preventive measure but also an effective management tool. Discover how exercise can be strategically incorporated to regulate blood sugar levels and enhance overall health.

Stress Management for Blood Sugar Control:

As stress directly influences blood sugar, this chapter will delve deeper into stress management techniques. Explore practices that align with your lifestyle, promoting both mental well-being and stable blood sugar levels.

By delving into the realm of monitoring and managing blood sugar levels, you are taking an active role in your health journey. This chapter equips you with practical tools and strategies to maintain balance, fostering a sense of empowerment and confidence as you navigate the path towards optimal well-being.

Chapter 5
Meal Planning and Recipes

In the intricate tapestry of blood sugar management, the role of nutrition cannot be overstated. Meal planning is a powerful tool that allows you to proactively shape your diet to support stable blood sugar levels. This chapter of "The Blood Sugar Solution" is your guide to crafting nutritious, balanced meals and exploring recipes that not only delight your taste buds but also contribute to your overall well-being.

Meal Plans for Blood Sugar Control

Balancing Macronutrients:

Explore meal plans that prioritize a balance of macronutrients—carbohydrates, proteins, and fats. This strategic combination helps regulate the release of glucose into the bloodstream, preventing sudden spikes and crashes in blood sugar levels.

14-Day Meal Plan for Blood Sugar Control

Day 1:

Breakfast:

- Scrambled eggs with spinach and mushrooms
- Whole grain toast
- Green tea

Lunch:

- Grilled chicken salad with mixed greens, cherry tomatoes, cucumbers, and balsamic vinaigrette
- Quinoa pilaf

Snack:

- Greek yogurt with sliced strawberries

Dinner:

- Baked salmon with lemon and dill
- Steamed broccoli
- Brown rice

Day 2:

Breakfast:

- Overnight oats with almond milk, chia seeds, and berries
- Boiled egg

Lunch:

- Turkey and avocado wrap with whole grain tortilla
- Carrot sticks with hummus

Snack:

- Handful of almonds

Dinner:

- Stir-fried tofu with bell peppers and snap peas
- Cauliflower rice

Day 3:

Breakfast:

- Whole grain pancakes with sugar-free syrup
- Fresh fruit salad

Lunch:

- Lentil soup
- Whole grain roll

Snack:

- Cottage cheese with cucumber slices

Dinner:

- Grilled shrimp skewers
- Roasted Brussels sprouts
- Quinoa

Day 4:

Breakfast:

- Greek yogurt parfait with granola and sliced bananas
- Green tea

Lunch:

- Spinach and feta stuffed chicken breast
- Steamed asparagus

Snack:

- Apple slices with almond butter

Dinner:

- Beef stir-fry with broccoli, bell peppers, and snow peas
- Brown rice

Day 5:

Breakfast:

- Vegetable omelette with spinach, tomatoes, and onions
- Whole grain toast

Lunch:

- Tuna salad with mixed greens, olives, and vinaigrette dressing
- Whole grain crackers

Snack:

- Sugar-free jello

Dinner:

- Baked cod with Mediterranean herbs
- Grilled zucchini
- Quinoa salad with cherry tomatoes and basil

Day 6:

Breakfast:

- Smoothie made with spinach, banana, almond milk, and protein powder
- Hard-boiled egg

Lunch:

- Grilled veggie wrap with hummus
- Kale chips

Snack:

- Celery sticks with peanut butter

Dinner:

- Turkey meatballs with marinara sauce
- Spaghetti squash
- Mixed green salad with vinaigrette

Day 7:

Breakfast:

- Whole grain toast with avocado
- Poached egg

Lunch:

- Chickpea salad with cucumbers, bell peppers, and lemon tahini dressing
- Whole grain pita

Snack:

- Cottage cheese with pineapple chunks

Dinner:

- Baked chicken breast with rosemary and garlic
- Roasted sweet potatoes
- Steamed green beans

Day 8:

Breakfast:

- Start your day with a protein-packed breakfast of scrambled eggs with spinach and mushrooms. This combination will keep you feeling full and satisfied throughout the morning. Pair it with a slice of whole grain toast for added fiber and energy.

Lunch:

- For lunch, enjoy a hearty grilled chicken salad loaded with mixed greens, cherry tomatoes, cucumbers, and a tangy balsamic vinaigrette dressing. Add a side of quinoa pilaf for complex carbohydrates and additional protein.

Snack:

- Snack on Greek yogurt topped with sliced strawberries. Greek yogurt is rich in protein and probiotics, which can help regulate blood sugar levels and improve gut health.

Dinner:

- For dinner, indulge in a delicious baked salmon seasoned with lemon and dill. Serve it alongside steamed broccoli and a serving of nutrient-rich brown rice for a balanced meal that's packed with flavor and nutrition.

Day 9:

Breakfast:

- Kickstart your morning with a satisfying bowl of overnight oats made with almond milk, chia seeds, and mixed berries. Overnight oats are a convenient and delicious way to fuel your body with fiber, protein, and antioxidants.

Lunch:

- Enjoy a turkey and avocado wrap made with a whole grain tortilla for lunch. Fill it with lean turkey breast, creamy avocado slices, and crunchy veggies like lettuce and tomato. Serve with a side of carrot sticks and hummus for added nutrients and fiber.

Snack:

- Keep hunger at bay with a handful of almonds. Almonds are a nutrient-dense snack that provides healthy fats, protein, and fiber to help stabilize blood sugar levels and keep you feeling full between meals.

Dinner:

- Prepare a flavorful stir-fry with tofu, bell peppers, and snap peas for dinner. Tofu is a great source of plant-based protein, while the colorful veggies add vitamins, minerals, and antioxidants to your meal. Serve over cauliflower rice for a low-carb alternative to traditional rice.

Day 10:

Breakfast:

- Treat yourself to a stack of whole grain pancakes topped with sugar-free syrup and a fresh fruit salad on the side. Whole grain pancakes are a delicious and nutritious breakfast option that provides complex carbohydrates for sustained energy.

Lunch:

- Warm up with a bowl of hearty lentil soup for lunch. Lentils are a good source of fiber and protein, which can help stabilize blood sugar levels and promote feelings of fullness. Pair the soup with a whole grain roll for a complete meal.

Snack:

- Enjoy a serving of cottage cheese with cucumber slices for a light and refreshing snack. Cottage cheese is high in protein and low in carbohydrates, making it an ideal option for blood sugar control.

Dinner:

- Treat yourself to grilled shrimp skewers served with roasted Brussels sprouts and a side of quinoa. Shrimp is a lean source of protein that pairs perfectly with the earthy flavors of Brussels sprouts and nutty quinoa for a satisfying and nutritious dinner.

Day 11:

Breakfast:

- Start your day with a protein-rich Greek yogurt parfait layered with granola and sliced bananas. Greek yogurt is an excellent source of protein and probiotics, while the bananas and granola add natural sweetness and crunch.

Lunch:

- Enjoy a spinach and feta stuffed chicken breast for lunch. This flavorful dish is packed with protein and vitamins, thanks to the combination of lean chicken breast and nutrient-rich spinach and feta cheese. Serve with a side of steamed asparagus for added fiber and antioxidants.

Snack:

- Satisfy your midday cravings with apple slices dipped in almond butter. Apples are high in fiber and antioxidants, while almond butter provides healthy fats and protein to keep you feeling satisfied until your next meal.

Dinner:

- Prepare a delicious beef stir-fry with broccoli, bell peppers, and snow peas for dinner. Beef is a good source of protein and iron, while the colorful veggies add vitamins, minerals, and fiber to your meal. Serve over brown rice for a hearty and nutritious dinner option.

Day 12:

Breakfast:

- Blend up a green smoothie made with spinach, banana, almond milk, and protein powder for a quick and nutritious breakfast on the go. Green smoothies are a great way to sneak in extra servings of vegetables and fruit while providing a boost of energy and essential nutrients.

Lunch:

- Enjoy a grilled veggie wrap filled with hummus for lunch. Load up a whole grain tortilla with grilled vegetables like zucchini, bell peppers, and onions, and spread a generous layer of hummus for added flavor and creaminess. Serve with a side of kale chips for a crunchy and satisfying meal.

Snack:

- Snack on celery sticks filled with peanut butter for a nutritious and satisfying snack. Celery is low in calories and high in fiber, while peanut butter provides healthy fats and protein to keep you feeling full and energized.

Dinner:

- Indulge in turkey meatballs with marinara sauce served over spaghetti squash for a lighter take on a classic Italian dish. Turkey meatballs are lower in fat than traditional beef meatballs but still pack plenty of flavor and protein. Pair with a mixed green salad dressed with vinaigrette for a balanced and delicious dinner.

Day 13:

Breakfast:

- Enjoy a simple yet satisfying breakfast of whole grain toast topped with creamy avocado and a poached egg. Avocado is rich in heart-healthy fats, while eggs provide protein and essential nutrients to start your day off on the right foot.

Lunch:

- Dig into a chickpea salad with cucumbers, bell peppers, and lemon tahini dressing for lunch. Chickpeas are high in fiber and protein, making them an excellent option for stabilizing blood sugar levels and promoting feelings of fullness. Pair with a whole grain pita for a satisfying and nutritious meal.

Snack:

- Treat yourself to cottage cheese topped with pineapple chunks for a sweet and creamy snack. Cottage cheese is high in protein and calcium, while pineapple adds natural sweetness and vitamin C to your snack.

Dinner:

- Prepare a flavorful baked chicken breast seasoned with rosemary and garlic for dinner. Serve alongside roasted sweet potatoes and steamed green beans for a balanced and nutritious meal that's packed with flavor and essential nutrients.

Day 14:

Breakfast:

- Start your day with a nutritious breakfast of scrambled eggs with spinach, tomatoes, and onions. This veggie-packed dish is rich in protein, vitamins, and minerals, making it an excellent choice for stabilizing blood sugar levels and promoting overall health.

Lunch:

- Enjoy a turkey and avocado wrap made with a whole grain tortilla for lunch. Fill it with lean turkey breast, creamy avocado slices, and crunchy veggies like lettuce and tomato. Serve with a side of carrot sticks and hummus for added nutrients and fiber.

Snack:

- Keep hunger at bay with a handful of almonds. Almonds are a nutrient-dense snack that provides healthy fats, protein, and fiber to help stabilize blood sugar levels and keep you feeling full between meals.

Dinner:

- Treat yourself to a delicious stir-fry made with tofu, bell peppers, and snap peas for dinner. Tofu is a plant-based source of protein that pairs perfectly with the vibrant flavors of the stir-fried veggies. Serve over cauliflower rice for a low-carb and nutritious twist on a classic dish.

Timing and Frequency of Meals:

Discover the significance of meal timing and frequency in blood sugar management. Explore meal plans that incorporate regular, well-timed meals and snacks to maintain steady energy levels throughout the day.

Healthy Recipes Tailored for Blood Sugar Balance

Breakfast Ideas:

Start your day right with nutritious breakfast options that set a positive tone for stable blood sugar levels. Explore recipes that combine complex carbohydrates, proteins, and healthy fats, providing sustained energy and satiety.

Lunch and Dinner Recipes:

Dive into a variety of lunch and dinner recipes that showcase a rich array of flavors while adhering to blood sugar-friendly principles. From vibrant salads to hearty, balanced main dishes, these recipes make mealtime a celebration of health and well-being.

Snack Options:

Discover satisfying snack options that curb cravings without causing undue spikes in blood sugar. From nutrient-dense smoothies to wholesome snack bars, these recipes offer both convenience and nutrition.

As you navigate the world of meal planning and recipes, consider this chapter as a compass guiding you towards a delicious and health-supportive journey. By incorporating these principles into your culinary repertoire, you'll not only savor the joy of flavorful meals but also contribute to the stability of your blood sugar levels. Get ready to embark on a culinary adventure that aligns with your health goals and enhances your overall well-being.

Recipes

Here are 10 recipes focused on blood sugar control:

Quinoa Salad with Chickpeas and Roasted Vegetables

Ingredients:

- 1 cup quinoa, rinsed
- 1 can chickpeas, drained and rinsed
- 1 red bell pepper, diced
- 1 yellow bell pepper, diced
- 1 zucchini, diced

- 1 small red onion, sliced
- 2 tablespoons olive oil
- 1 teaspoon dried oregano
- Salt and pepper to taste
- Juice of 1 lemon
- 2 tablespoons chopped fresh parsley

Directions:

- Set oven temperature to 400°F, or 200°C.
- Combine the red onion, bell peppers, zucchini, and chickpeas in a big bowl along with the olive oil, oregano, salt, and pepper.
- After spreading them out on a baking sheet, roast the vegetables in a preheated oven for 20 to 25 minutes, or until they are soft and beginning to brown.
- As you wait, prepare the quinoa per the directions on the package.
- Place the cooked quinoa and the roasted veggies in a large mixing basin.
- Pour the lemon juice over the salad and mix everything together.
- Before serving, garnish with fresh parsley.

Nutritional Information (per serving):

- Calories: 321

- Protein: 9g

- Carbohydrates: 51g

- Fiber: 9g

- Fat: 7g

Baked Salmon with Asparagus and Lemon

Ingredients:

- 4 salmon fillets

- 1 bunch asparagus, trimmed

- 2 tablespoons olive oil

- 2 cloves garlic, minced

- 1 lemon, sliced

- Salt and pepper to taste

- Fresh dill for garnish (optional)

Directions:

- Set oven temperature to 400°F, or 200°C.

- Arrange the asparagus and salmon fillets on a parchment paper-lined baking sheet.

- Pour some olive oil on the asparagus and fish. Evenly distribute the salt, pepper, and minced garlic on top.

- Top each salmon fillet with a slice of lemon.

- Bake the salmon for 12 to 15 minutes, or until it is cooked through and flake readily with a fork, in an oven that has been warmed.

- If preferred, garnish with fresh dill prior to serving.

Nutritional Information (per serving):

- Calories: 302

- Protein: 31g

- Carbohydrates: 6g

- Fiber: 3g

- Fat: 19g

Turkey and Vegetable Stir-Fry

Ingredients:

- 1 lb turkey breast, thinly sliced

- 2 cups mixed vegetables (bell peppers, broccoli, snap peas, carrots)

- 2 tablespoons low-sodium soy sauce

- 1 tablespoon sesame oil

- 2 cloves garlic, minced

- 1 teaspoon ginger, grated

- 2 green onions, sliced

- Cooked brown rice for serving

Directions:

- In a large skillet or wok, heat the sesame oil over medium-high heat.
- Stir-fry the grated ginger and minced garlic for a minute or until fragrant.
- Add the turkey slices and heat for 5 to 7 minutes, or until browned and cooked through.
- Stir-fry the mixed vegetables in the skillet for a further three to four minutes, or until they are crisp-tender.
- Add sliced green onions and low-sodium soy sauce and stir.
- After the brown rice has cooked, serve the stir-fry.

Nutritional Information (per serving without rice):

- Calories: 252
- Protein: 31g
- Carbohydrates: 11g
- Fiber: 4g
- Fat: 8g

Greek Yogurt Parfait

Ingredients:

- 1 cup Greek yogurt

- 1/2 cup mixed berries (strawberries, blueberries, raspberries)

- 1/4 cup granola (look for low-sugar options)

- 1 tablespoon honey (optional)

Directions:

- Arrange Greek yogurt, granola, and mixed berries in a glass or bowl.

- If desired, drizzle honey over the top.

- If preparing several servings, repeat layering.

- Serve right away or put in the fridge until you're ready to eat.

Nutritional Information (per serving):

- Calories: 252

- Protein: 19g

- Carbohydrates: 34g

- Fiber: 6g

- Fat: 7g

Veggie Egg Muffins

Ingredients:

- 6 eggs

- 1 cup mixed vegetables (bell peppers, spinach, onions)
- Salt and pepper to taste
- Cooking spray

Directions:

- Set the oven's temperature to 175°C/350°F. Put cooking spray to a muffin tin and grease it.
- Whisk the eggs, salt, and pepper in a mixing bowl.
- Add mixed vegetables and stir until thoroughly blended.
- Fill each cup of the muffin tin approximately 3/4 of the way to the top with the egg and veggie mixture.
- Bake for 20 to 25 minutes in a preheated oven, or until the tops of the egg muffins are gently brown and set.
- Before taking the muffins out of the tin, let them cool somewhat.
- Serve warm or keep chilled for up to 4 days in an airtight container.

Nutritional Information (per serving - 2 muffins):

- Calories: 161
- Protein: 13g

- Carbohydrates: 6g
- Fiber: 3g
- Fat: 11g

Chicken and Vegetable Skewers

Ingredients:

- 1 lb boneless, skinless chicken breast, cut into cubes
- 2 bell peppers, cut into chunks
- 1 red onion, cut into chunks
- 1 zucchini, sliced
- 2 tablespoons olive oil
- 1 teaspoon garlic powder
- 1 teaspoon paprika
- Salt and pepper to taste

Directions:

- Set the grill's temperature to medium-high.
- Toss the veggies and chicken cubes in a bowl with olive oil, salt, pepper, paprika, and garlic powder until well covered.
- On skewers, alternate layers of chicken and vegetables are threaded.

- Cook the skewers for 10 to 12 minutes, rotating them halfway through, or until the vegetables are soft and the chicken is cooked through.
- If preferred, serve the freshly grilled skewers hot with brown rice or a side salad.

Nutritional Information (per serving):

- Calories: 252
- Protein: 26g
- Carbohydrates: 11g
- Fiber: 4g
- Fat: 13g

Lentil Soup

Ingredients:

- 1 cup dried green lentils, rinsed
- 4 cups low-sodium vegetable broth
- 1 onion, chopped
- 2 carrots, chopped
- 2 celery stalks, chopped
- 2 cloves garlic, minced
- 1 teaspoon dried thyme
- 1 bay leaf
- Salt and pepper to taste

- Fresh parsley for garnish

Directions:

- Warm up the olive oil in a big pot over medium heat. Cook the chopped onion, carrots, celery, and garlic for approximately five minutes, or until they are tender.
- Add the dried lentils, bay leaf, dried thyme, vegetable broth, salt, and pepper and stir.
- After bringing the soup to a boil, lower the heat, and simmer it for 20 to 25 minutes, or until the lentils are soft.
- Take out and dispose of the bay leaf from the soup.
- Before serving, ladle the soup into dishes and sprinkle with fresh parsley.

Nutritional Information (per serving):

- Calories: 221
- Protein: 15g
- Carbohydrates: 41g
- Fiber: 17g
- Fat: 2g

Spinach and Feta Stuffed Chicken Breast

Ingredients:

- 4 boneless, skinless chicken breasts
- 2 cups fresh spinach leaves
- 1/2 cup crumbled feta cheese
- 2 cloves garlic, minced
- 1 teaspoon dried oregano
- Salt and pepper to taste
- Cooking spray

Directions:

- Turn the oven on to 375°F, or 190°C. Use cooking spray to grease a baking dish.
- To make a pocket, butterfly each chicken breast by cutting a horizontal cut in the middle, leaving one edge uncut.
- Add the spinach, feta cheese, dried oregano, minced garlic, salt, and pepper to a mixing bowl.
- Place a toothpick into the opening of each chicken breast after stuffing it with the spinach and feta mixture.
- Stuff the chicken breasts into the baking dish that has been prepared.

- Bake for 25 to 30 minutes in a preheated oven, or until the chicken is thoroughly cooked and the juices are clear.

- Take off the toothpicks prior to serving.

Nutritional Information (per serving):

- Calories: 282

- Protein: 41g

- Carbohydrates: 3g

- Fiber: 2g

- Fat: 13g

Tuna Salad Lettuce Wraps

Ingredients:

- 2 cans tuna, drained

- 1/4 cup Greek yogurt

- 1/4 cup diced celery

- 1/4 cup diced red onion

- 1 tablespoon lemon juice

- 1 teaspoon Dijon mustard

- Salt and pepper to taste

- Lettuce leaves for wrapping

Directions:

- Drained tuna, Greek yogurt, diced red onion, diced celery, lemon juice, Dijon mustard, salt, and pepper should all be combined in a mixing dish.

- Mix thoroughly to ensure that the dressing coats the tuna evenly.

- Place a spoonful of tuna salad onto each lettuce leaf, wrap, and, if necessary, fasten with toothpicks.

- Serve lettuce wraps with tuna salad for a light and energizing dinner or snack.

Nutritional Information (per serving):

- Calories: 182
- Protein: 33g
- Carbohydrates: 5g
- Fiber: 2g
- Fat: 5g

Berry Smoothie Bowl

Ingredients:

- 1 cup mixed berries (strawberries, blueberries, raspberries)
- 1/2 cup Greek yogurt
- 1/4 cup almond milk
- 1 tablespoon chia seeds

- 1 tablespoon honey (optional)
- Toppings: sliced bananas, granola, shredded coconut

Directions:

- Blend together mixed berries, honey, chia seeds, Greek yogurt, and almond milk in a blender (if using).
- To get the right consistency, add extra almond milk if necessary and blend until smooth and creamy.
- After transferring the smoothie into a bowl, garnish it with shredded coconut, granola, and banana slices.
- Present right away and savour with a spoon.

Nutritional Information (per serving):

- Calories: 252
- Protein: 13g
- Carbohydrates: 36g
- Fiber: 9g
- Fat: 8g

Chapter 6
Overcoming Challenges

Embarking on the journey to balance blood sugar is a commendable endeavor, yet it's not without its share of challenges. In this chapter, we'll explore common hurdles faced on the path to optimal blood sugar levels and equip you with practical strategies to overcome them. From managing sugar cravings to navigating social events, this chapter is your guide to triumphing over challenges and maintaining your commitment to a balanced and vibrant life.

Dealing with Sugar Cravings

Understanding Cravings:

Delve into the science behind sugar cravings—why they occur and how they can impact blood sugar levels. Recognizing the root causes is the first step in developing effective strategies to manage and overcome these cravings.

Healthy Alternatives:

Explore a palette of healthy alternatives to satisfy your sweet tooth without compromising your blood sugar goals. From naturally sweet fruits to mindful indulgences, discover options that align with your dietary preferences and health objectives.

Dining Out Strategies

Making Informed Choices:

Dining out doesn't have to be a challenge for blood sugar management. Learn how to make informed choices when perusing restaurant menus, opting for options that are not only delicious but also supportive of stable blood sugar levels.

Navigating Restaurant Challenges:

From portion control to hidden sugars, uncover strategies for navigating common challenges encountered when dining out. These insights empower you to enjoy restaurant experiences while prioritizing your health goals.

Navigating Social Events and Holidays

Communication and Planning:

Social events and holidays often revolve around food, presenting unique challenges for blood sugar management. Discover effective communication strategies and proactive planning techniques to navigate these occasions with confidence.

Mindful Celebration:

Celebrating special occasions can coexist with your commitment to blood sugar balance. Explore ways to make mindful choices during festivities, ensuring that you not only enjoy the moment but also prioritize your health.

As you delve into the strategies for overcoming challenges, remember that setbacks are a natural part of any journey. The key lies in resilience, adaptability, and the knowledge that each challenge conquered is a step closer to sustained well-being. Consider this chapter as your companion in facing obstacles head-on, arming you with the tools to triumph over challenges and continue your pursuit of optimal blood sugar balance.

Chapter 7

Long-Term Health and Wellness

In the ever-evolving journey of blood sugar management, the focus extends beyond immediate challenges to the enduring goal of long-term health and wellness. This chapter delves into the profound impact that sustained blood sugar balance can have on your overall health. As we explore preventive measures for conditions like Type 2 diabetes and delve into the relationship between blood sugar and weight management, envision a future where your commitment to well-being yields lasting benefits.

Prevention of Type 2 Diabetes

Understanding Type 2 Diabetes Risk Factors:

Delve into the risk factors associated with Type 2 diabetes and how maintaining optimal blood sugar levels can serve as a powerful preventive measure. By addressing modifiable risk factors, you empower yourself to proactively reduce the likelihood of developing this chronic condition.

Lifestyle Strategies for Prevention:

Explore lifestyle strategies that go beyond immediate blood sugar management, fostering habits that contribute to the prevention of Type 2 diabetes. From sustained physical activity to mindful dietary choices, these strategies form the foundation of a proactive and preventive approach to long-term health.

Blood Sugar Solution for Weight Management

The Interconnection of Blood Sugar and Weight:

Uncover the intricate relationship between blood sugar levels and weight management. Understand how the two interplays, influencing each other, and explore strategies to achieve a healthy weight that supports overall well-being.

Lifestyle Habits for Sustainable Weight Management:

Beyond fad diets and temporary solutions, embrace lifestyle habits that promote sustainable weight management. Discover the synergy between balanced blood sugar levels, nutritious food choices, and regular physical activity in achieving and maintaining a healthy weight.

Impact on Overall Health and Well-Being

Beyond Blood Sugar: Holistic Health Benefits:

Acknowledge the ripple effect of blood sugar balance on overall health. From enhanced energy levels to improved mood and cognitive function, discover the holistic health benefits that extend beyond the immediate focus on blood sugar.

Thriving in Well-Being:

Envision a future where your commitment to long-term health and wellness blossoms into a state of thriving well-being. By consistently adopting the principles of The Blood Sugar Solution, you set the stage for a life marked by vitality, resilience, and enduring health.

As you absorb the insights in this chapter, recognize that your journey is not only about managing blood sugar but about cultivating a life of sustained well-being. The choices you make today echo into the future, creating a legacy of health and vitality that extends far beyond blood sugar management alone. Consider this chapter as your roadmap to a future where optimal health becomes a constant companion on your life's journey.

Chapter 8
Real-Life Success Stories

As we traverse the path of blood sugar management together, it's inspiring and motivating to hear the stories of individuals who have faced similar challenges and triumphed on their journey to optimal well-being. In this chapter, we'll dive into real-life success stories—compelling narratives of individuals who have embraced The Blood Sugar Solution and witnessed transformative changes in their health. These stories serve as beacons of hope, illustrating that with commitment, knowledge, and perseverance, achieving balanced blood sugar levels is not only possible but also a transformative and empowering experience.

Personal Journeys to Blood Sugar Control

Overcoming Challenges:

Meet individuals who have faced diverse challenges in their blood sugar management journey. From battling sugar cravings to navigating lifestyle changes, these stories highlight the resilience and determination required to overcome obstacles and achieve lasting success.

Triumphs in Lifestyle Transformation:

Explore how these individuals embraced The Blood Sugar Solution Lifestyle, incorporating dietary changes, regular exercise, and stress management into their daily routines. Their triumphs serve as testaments to the power of sustainable lifestyle changes in achieving and maintaining balanced blood sugar levels.

Lessons Learned and Inspirational Narratives

Navigating Setbacks:

Blood sugar management is a dynamic process, and setbacks are a natural part of the journey. Discover how individuals faced and navigated setbacks, using them as opportunities for growth and learning rather than obstacles.

Sustainable Lifestyle Changes:

Hear firsthand about the sustainable lifestyle changes which individuals incorporated into their lives. From mindful eating practices to regular physical activity, these narratives emphasize the importance of holistic approaches for long-term success.

Encouragement for Your Journey

Shared Insights and Wisdom:

The stories in this chapter not only share personal victories but also offer insights and wisdom gained through firsthand experience. Discover pearls of knowledge that may resonate with your own journey and serve as guidance for overcoming challenges.

Empowering Others:

Many individuals who have successfully managed their blood sugar levels find fulfillment in empowering others on a similar path. Explore how these success stories become catalysts for positive change, inspiring and supporting others in their pursuit of optimal health.

As you immerse yourself in these real-life success stories, remember that each journey is unique. Whether you're at the beginning of your blood sugar management adventure or navigating challenges along the way, these stories are a source of inspiration, encouragement, and proof that lasting success is achievable. Consider this chapter as a celebration of the resilience of the human spirit and a testament to the transformative power of The Blood Sugar Solution.

Chapter 9

Resources for Further Support

On your journey toward optimal blood sugar levels and lasting well-being, access to reliable resources and ongoing support is invaluable. This chapter serves as a comprehensive guide, directing you to a variety of tools, communities, and experts that can enhance your understanding, provide additional insights, and offer ongoing encouragement. Whether you prefer books, workshops, online communities, or professional guidance, these resources are designed to complement and support your individual path to balanced blood sugar and sustained health.

Books and Reading Materials

In-Depth Knowledge:

Explore a curated list of books that delve into the science, lifestyle strategies, and personal stories related to blood sugar management. These resources provide in-depth knowledge and diverse perspectives, empowering you to further understand and navigate your journey.

Cookbooks for Balanced Eating:

Discover cookbooks specifically tailored to support balanced blood sugar levels. These resources offer a wealth of delicious recipes and meal ideas that align with the principles of The Blood Sugar Solution, making healthy eating an enjoyable and flavorful experience.

Workshops and Seminars

Interactive Learning:

Engage in interactive learning experiences through workshops and seminars. These resources provide opportunities to deepen your understanding, ask questions, and connect with experts and fellow participants on a similar journey. Workshops can cover a range of topics, from meal planning to stress management.

Local and Online Events:

Stay informed about local and online events focused on blood sugar management and overall well-being. Participating in events allows you to access the latest information, network with like-minded individuals, and gain practical insights from experts in the field.

Online Communities and Forums

Peer Support:

Connect with others on a similar journey through online communities and forums. Share your experiences, learn from others, and find inspiration and encouragement from a supportive community. These platforms provide a space to ask questions, celebrate victories, and navigate challenges together.

Expert Guidance:

Some online communities feature expert-led discussions and Q&A sessions. Engage with healthcare professionals, nutritionists, and wellness experts who can offer personalized advice, answer specific questions, and provide evidence-based insights to further guide your blood sugar management journey.

Professional Guidance

Nutritional Counseling:

Consider seeking the guidance of a registered dietitian or nutritionist specializing in blood sugar management. Personalized nutritional counseling can provide tailored advice, meal planning support, and ongoing guidance to address your specific needs and goals.

Medical Professionals:

Work in collaboration with your healthcare team, including your primary care physician and endocrinologist. Regular check-ups, blood tests, and open communication with your healthcare providers are crucial components of a comprehensive approach to blood sugar management.

As you explore these resources, remember that each individual's journey is unique. Tailor your approach based on your preferences, needs, and lifestyle. The aim is not only to manage blood sugar levels effectively but also to foster a sense of empowerment and well-being. Consider this chapter as your compass, guiding you toward the diverse and supportive resources available to enhance your journey towards balanced blood sugar and lasting health.

Chapter 10
Embracing a Life of Balanced Blood Sugar

As we reach the conclusion of "The Blood Sugar Solution," take a moment to reflect on the journey you've undertaken, the knowledge you've gained, and the transformative steps you've implemented toward balanced blood sugar and lasting well-being. This concluding chapter serves as a bridge between the insights you've gathered and the ongoing journey that lies ahead. Let's encapsulate the key points, provide encouragement, and express wishes for a future marked by vitality, health, and fulfillment.

Recap of Key Points

Understanding Blood Sugar:

Reflect on the foundational knowledge gained about blood sugar—its role in the body, the factors influencing its balance, and the profound impact it has on overall health.

Lifestyle Strategies:

Revisit the lifestyle strategies introduced throughout the book, from dietary guidelines and physical activity to stress management and sustained well-being. Consider how these strategies have become integral components of your daily life.

Success Stories and Inspiration:

Celebrate the real-life success stories shared in Chapter 8, recognizing the resilience, commitment, and transformative power of individuals who have embraced The Blood Sugar Solution.

Encouragement for the Journey Ahead

Your Personal Empowerment:

Recognize your role as the captain of your health journey. Embrace the empowerment that comes with understanding and actively managing your blood sugar levels.

Resilience in the Face of Challenges:

Acknowledge that challenges are a natural part of any journey. Remember the insights shared in Chapter 7 on overcoming challenges, and let each obstacle be an opportunity for growth and adaptation.

Sustainable Lifestyle Choices:

Reaffirm your commitment to sustainable lifestyle choices. These choices are not temporary measures but enduring pillars that support your journey to optimal health.

Wishing You a Happy and Fulfilling Future

Vibrant Health and Well-Being:

Envision a future marked by vibrant health, sustained well-being, and a sense of fulfillment. Your commitment to balanced blood sugar is not just about managing a condition—it's about embracing a holistic and fulfilling life.

Continued Learning and Growth:

Embrace the spirit of lifelong learning and growth. Stay curious, explore new insights, and remain open to evolving strategies that support your well-being.

Community and Support:

Remember the diverse resources introduced in the previous Chapter. Leverage the support of communities, professionals, and ongoing educational opportunities to enrich your journey.

As you turn the final pages of "The Blood Sugar Solution," envision a future where optimal health is not a destination but a continuous journey. Your commitment to balanced blood sugar is a testament to your dedication to a life of vitality and well-being. Here's to your ongoing success, resilience in the face of challenges, and the fulfillment of a life well-lived. May your path be marked by health, happiness, and a sense of purpose. Cheers to the journey ahead!

Conclusion

"The Solution for Blood Sugar" stands as a beacon of hope and empowerment for individuals seeking to take control of their health and well-being in the face of blood sugar challenges. Throughout the pages of this comprehensive guide, we have delved deep into the intricate complexities of blood sugar management, offering a wealth of practical knowledge, evidence-based strategies, and insightful advice to support you on your journey toward achieving optimal health.

In a world inundated with misinformation and confusion surrounding blood sugar control, this book serves as a trusted companion, providing clarity, guidance, and actionable steps to navigate the intricacies of managing blood sugar levels effectively. From understanding the physiological mechanisms that regulate blood sugar to implementing practical lifestyle interventions, each chapter is meticulously crafted to empower you with the tools and knowledge needed to make informed decisions about your health.

Central to our approach is the recognition that blood sugar management is not merely about monitoring numbers on a glucose meter, but rather, it encompasses a holistic approach to health that encompasses nutrition, physical activity, stress management, sleep hygiene, and mindful living. By addressing these interconnected facets of well-being, we aim to equip you with a comprehensive toolkit for promoting stable blood sugar levels and enhancing overall vitality.

Throughout the journey outlined in these pages, we have explored the transformative power of nutrition as a cornerstone of blood sugar control. From embracing whole, nutrient-dense foods to making mindful choices about carbohydrate intake, readers are empowered to cultivate a nourishing diet that supports stable blood sugar levels and promotes long-term health.

Moreover, we have delved into the profound impact of physical activity on blood sugar regulation, highlighting the importance of regular exercise in improving insulin sensitivity, enhancing glucose uptake, and promoting cardiovascular health. Whether it's engaging in aerobic activities, strength training, or yoga, incorporating movement into your daily routine is essential for achieving optimal blood sugar control and overall well-being.

In addition to dietary and lifestyle interventions, "The Solution for Blood Sugar" underscores the critical role of stress management and emotional well-being in blood sugar control. Through mindfulness practices, relaxation techniques, and cultivating a supportive social network, readers are encouraged to foster resilience in the face of life's challenges, thereby reducing the detrimental effects of stress on blood sugar levels and overall health.

The importance of quality sleep in blood sugar regulation, highlighting the profound impact of sleep deprivation on insulin sensitivity, glucose metabolism, and appetite regulation. By prioritizing restorative sleep hygiene practices and establishing healthy sleep habits, readers can optimize their body's ability to regulate blood sugar levels and support overall health and vitality.

As we bring this journey to a close, it is essential to acknowledge that achieving optimal blood sugar control is not a destination but rather a lifelong journey characterized by commitment, persistence, and resilience. While the road may be fraught with challenges and setbacks, each obstacle presents an opportunity for growth, learning, and self-discovery.

In closing, "The Solution for Blood Sugar" is more than just a book; it is a beacon of hope, empowerment, and transformation for individuals seeking to reclaim their health and vitality in the face of blood sugar challenges. May the insights, strategies, and inspiration shared within these pages serve as a guiding light on your journey toward achieving optimal blood sugar control and embracing a life of vibrant health and well-being.

www.ingramcontent.com/pod-product-compliance
Lightning Source LLC
Chambersburg PA
CBHW051656250726
48653CB00007B/2693